Flexible Dieting Maximum Results

BY CHRIS COLE

The Ultimate Guide On How Flexible Dieting Can Build A Bigger, Leaner and Stronger You!

Second Edition

I0427976

Chris Cole

Copyright

Flexible Dieting Maximum Results: The Ultimate Guide On How Flexible Dieting Can Build A Bigger, Leaner and Stronger You!
Second Edition – May 2015
© Copyright 2015 by Chris Cole- All rights reserved.

Legal Notice

Disclaimer Notice

Table of Contents

Table of Contents 4

Introduction.. 6

Chapter 1: Understanding Flexible
     Dieting 8

Chapter 2: Common Misconceptions
     about Flexible Dieting 11

Chapter 3: Perks of Flexible Dieting 13

Chapter 4: Nutrients and Calories: The
     Science Behind Muscle
     Growth 17

Chapter 5: Beginner's Guide to Flexible
     Dieting 20

Chapter 6: Flexible Dieting is All You
     Need!... 23

Chapter 7: Why Protein Is So Important 26

Chapter 8: The Case Against Processed
     Foods 30

Chapter 9: Weight Loss And Fat Loss
     Are Different 34

Chapter 10: Changing Your Attitude
     Towards Dieting 36

Chapter 11: The Right Approach To Free
     Meals And Structured Re-
     feeds 40

Chapter 12: Taking a Dieting Break.................... 47

Chapter 13: Why Eating Lower Fat Content Matters **52**

Chapter 14: Carbohydrates and Insulin **58**

Chapter 15: Why Flexible Dieting Works When Other Diets Fail **62**

Conclusion **67**

Preview of My Other Books **68**

Introduction

Flexible dieting does what it says on the tin – it's a totally flexible system of weight loss and weight maintenance, where you can eat what you want to, as long as your food choices hit your macro nutrient requirements. That's proteins, carbohydrates and fats, if you're wondering. The concept is also called 'If it fits your macro (IIFYM), and although the macro nutrient bit is the most important part of flexible dieting, calories count too, because any diet depends on calorie deficit to lose weight. Whatever name your chosen diet rejoices in, the fact remains that to lose one pound in weight, you need to take in 3,500 less calories than your body needs for healthy function. There's no getting away from that.

Where flexible dieting wins over other diets is by placing more choice in the hands of the dieter. You can choose what you want to eat, rather than building your diet around cutting out forbidden foods, which always seem more desirable if you know you can't have them. There's an old saying that 'Forbidden fruits taste sweeter,' and it's certainly true about diets. Even if you didn't enjoy a particular food in your pre diet days, once it's off limits, you're likely to crave it.

Flexible dieting puts an end to forbidden foods, and an end to cravings, so it's a healthy eating plan you can live with. And if you're going to lose weight and keep it off, you will need to live with it. This book aims to teach you everything you need to know about flexible dieting, so you can build a leaner and stronger you.

I hope you get as much value from it as I have and trust you get real value from my book. I hope you enjoy it.

Chapter 1: Understanding Flexible Dieting

One of the most reverberating yet clichéd beliefs when it comes to food habits and health is that physical fitness comes with a catch, a very big one, and that is having to say no to your favorite foods. But what if you could still meet your fitness goals without having to refuse a piece of chocolate cake at your friend's birthday party? Or decline an invitation to go to a pizzeria with your co-workers? But no, no, broccoli is healthy, pizza is not. This was the common belief until the brilliance of flexible dieting began manifesting itself in the world of nutrition and health. Let's see what it is.

Flexible Dieting is a nutritional concept which believes in monitoring the intake of food in terms of macronutrients (carbohydrates, proteins and fats) irrespective of the quality of food, as an aid to weight loss or gain. It stems from the fact that food, be it healthy or junk, is basically a storehouse of macronutrients which are metabolized by the body in the same way, regardless of their source. This is in contrast to a traditional diet where each food is measured for its total calories and termed as healthy or unhealthy.

There is a certain value of each macronutrient required by a particular person per day. This value differs from person to person depending on a variety of factors like age, gender, lifestyle etc. Now, the key is to eat food so as to meet this macronutrient target. A gram of each macronutrient has a certain calorie value assigned to it. A flexible dieter overlooks the ratio of calories and focuses on nutrients. This is a smarter choice in varying body composition because it ensures a healthy distribution of the right amount of each nutrient. At the end of the day, what matters is whether the nutrient target has been achieved, and not whether it came from a salad or a burger.

Flexible dieting, also called 'If It Fits Your Macros' (IIFYM) is not really a diet. It is more of a conscious choice by a person to eat according to his or her needs. The widespread acceptance of this method as a proven weight loss/gain technique has been a recent phenomenon even though the concept behind it has been prevailing in the body building industry for quite some time. Bland, tasteless food is what comes under the label of healthy or 'clean' food which is prescribed by most fitness experts to anyone cautious about their health.

The monotonous routine of the same food taken at specific intervals is bound to make anyone feel miserable after some time. This is in addition to the social exclusion it creates because a person who strictly adheres to such a strict diet cannot go to most social gatherings and enjoy the food that is available. This creates feelings of intense deprivation and the person quits the whole thing before achieving his goals. On the other hand, flexible dieting is not an abrupt drop in calorie intake by cutting down almost all of the tasty foods, but a steady, sustained way of eating which meets the daily requirement of each nutrient from a diet comprising of a bulk of healthy food along with a permitted amount of tasty, junk food from time to time.

Now it's necessary to examine in detail the advantages of choosing the flexible dieting method, and to discover how it helps in achieving the desired body composition goals without the hassle and feelings of deprivation often associated with traditional exclusion diets.

Chapter 2: Common Misconceptions about Flexible Dieting

Parallel to the spread of flexible dieting are the various misunderstandings regarding its basic facts. It is essential to know what is true and what is false before you embark on this journey to physical fitness. There are three important myths that circulate around this concept, and it's necessary to examine those and put the record straight.

What exactly is clean eating when it comes to flexible dieting?

Clean food, in its most basic sense, refers to healthy food. It is food in its most natural, low calorie state prescribed in the case of diets. It is a common mistake in believing that the notion of eating clean is prevalent in flexible dieting. Anthony Collova, owner of www.iifym.com defines clean food with regard to flexible dieting as "any single ingredient food item." It could be anything- butter, rice or fruits. Flexible dieting does not care whether the food is unhealthy, fatty, organic or vegan. Every single ingredient item is a clean food with its specific constitution of macronutrients. All you have to do is stick within your macronutrient limit and not exceed it.

Flexible dieting lets you eat as much junk food as you want.

This is the most common misconception regarding flexible dieting, and it originated from those practitioners who do not abstain from junk food. This led to the myth that flexible dieting is all about eating junk food and still managing the perfect body. Wrong! Although it is true that flexible dieting lets you eat any type of food you want, it does not necessarily mean endless amounts of junk food. It is impossible to get all the required macro nutrients from a diet comprising purely of junk food. Therefore, most flexible dieters follow a healthy diet along with a permitted amount of unhealthy food. The key point is to hit the required quantity of each macronutrient per day, and that can come from clean food or junk food.

Flexible dieting is unhealthy

The notion of eating only clean food compared to eating anything you want sounds like the obvious smart choice but it is not. Flexible dieting is consuming a highly nutritional diet comprising of vegetables, fruits and whole grains, incorporating a few 'naughty but nice' delicacies at certain times. It is difficult to get the required amount of carbohydrates solely from a diet of organic vegetables. An average body does require low nutrient food at times in order to take in the required number of calories for healthy physical function. Therefore, it is healthier to eat everything in moderation rather than follow stringent diet plans which involve placing all your favorite foods off limits.

Chapter 3: Perks of Flexible Dieting

The concept of flexible dieting, erstwhile considered as a form of placebo in physical fitness, has slowly come to be recognized and accepted as a proven method of fitness achievement. However, as different fitness methods and conflicting opinions on each one of them abound in every corner of the fitness industry, the question of why people should choose flexible eating over any other means, say clean eating, is valid. There are a multitude of reasons that have tipped the scales in favor of flexible dieting. Here is a brief insight on the reasons to opt for an IIFYM diet.

Freedom in food choices

This is the biggest advantage of following a flexible diet- the freedom to eat anything you want, in lieu of repeating the same food day after day. You never find a flexible dieter immensely craving for a certain food because he is never restricted from having it. Once the macro nutrient requirement is accounted for, the rest of the calories can be compensated by eating anything that you wish, as long as it does not go over the set limit. Most flexible dieters therefore consume a bulk of healthy food and if they feel like it, a small treat of junk food which has been adjusted to fit into the daily calorie requirement. It can be met according to a person's own choice of meal timings or frequency of meals and not according to any laid down rules. Also, you can have the same eating behavior on weekends as on weekdays, unlike clean eating, when you completely abstain from junk food at some point and then look forward to having your cheat meals where you might possibly cram down unhealthy amounts of junk food to compensate for your deprivation.

No social isolation

A major drawback of clean eating is the social exclusion it creates in a person. Since only very few number of foods are designated as healthy, followers of the diet find themselves shying away from most social gatherings because the food provided is off limits to them. This adds to the misery created from not being able to eat the food you like and the practice of dieting becomes a period of suffering. Instead of becoming a social outcast, flexibility in diet lets you go out and enjoy any type of food, as long as the intake is kept in track.

Rules out eating disorders

The main reason why normal diets fail is because the feeling of deprivation creates eating disorders in a person, that is, once an opportunity arises, he or she finds himself in a binging spree followed by days of intense exercise, calorie counting and guilt. He is not able to carry on emotionally or physically in a healthy way because every food appears as good or bad and even a slight deviation from the prescribed path affects the overall wellbeing of the person. However, in case of flexibility, a person can include different types of food in his diet on a regular basis. Therefore he does not eat more than he is supposed, and won't get himself stressed out about having overindulged at some point – which is inevitable when you forbid foods and drastically restrict calories.

Flexible dieting is effective

Regulating the ratio of macronutrients without giving up an entire class of food does indeed help one achieve their fitness goals, be it weight loss or gaining leaner muscles. Since flexible dieting necessitates the need to track calorie values, this creates a better awareness of the body's nutrient requirements and meeting specifically those requirements without leaving room for additional calorie storage as fat. The lack of food deprivation helps a person on a holistic level which makes it even more effective in the long run.

Flexible dieting is sustainable

Clean eating may help one achieve short term weight loss goals, but to consistently follow its strict dietary rules becomes increasingly difficult as time goes by. Inevitably, once the goal has been met, the person resorts back to his original lifestyle of eating everything or in most cases, overeating. This nullifies any improvement in fitness which may have been created from a period of dieting. On the other hand, the lack of eating regulations makes flexible dieting seem just like a normal, healthier habit. Also, the increased knowledge of one's own food requirements makes it an easy task to continue following it. That is, flexible dieting is for long term. It just creates a healthier shift in a person's food habits which gets sustained as a part of a healthy lifestyle.

Flexibility in meal timings

With flexible dieting, you don't have to stick to specific food at particular times of the day. Meal frequency can be increased or decreased as per your bodily demands or your own preferences. You don't have to panic if you missed one of your daily meals, because you can easily make up for it by including the required nutrients in any other meal of the day. As long as you hit your daily macro ratios, the number of meals it took to achieve those values is irrelevant. So if you're a 'one meal a day' person, you can frame flexible dieting to reflect your preferences.

Chapter 4: Nutrients and Calories: The Science Behind Muscle Growth

Once you have started counting your macro nutrients rather than calories, it becomes easier to control your body weight by effective manipulation of nutrients. In order to obtain the full potential of flexible eating in achieving a better physique, it is important to know what is meant by muscle growth and how it is affected by the food you eat.

Nutrients are a prerequisite for growth and metabolism in the body. They can be macronutrients like proteins, carbohydrates and fats which are required in large amounts or micro nutrients like vitamins and minerals which are required in smaller amounts. Other than this, fibers are required for removing the waste byproducts created in the body during muscle growth. Thus, fiber aids in weight loss as these wastes can be reabsorbed by the body if they remain inside for long. Vegetables are a good source of fiber and by cleaning out the intestines, fiber content also allows for the effective absorption of nutrients.

In order to lose weight, your calorie intake must be lesser than the energy that you spend, and to gain weight, it must be more than the expended energy. This simple equation of energy consumed vs. energy expended can be used to add bulk, shed or maintain body weight. A calorie is a calorie irrespective of its macro nutrient composition. Strict dieters who restrict their calorie intake may lose weight, but this is just an even distribution of muscles and fat and not a healthy muscle growth. To gain a pound of muscle, around 2,800 calories are required per day, every day for a week, and in order to promote muscle growth all required nutrients are to be included in the diet. Thus, only by regulating daily calorie intake and hitting each macro nutrient target can one bring about the desired changes in the body's appearance.

When there is a demand for calories, the stored fat in the body gets broken down to release energy. This energy can be released and stored in muscle tissues during a bout of starvation and availability of the required nutrients will greatly promote muscle growth during this period. Muscle growth may occur in the absence of calories for beginners, but in the absence of nutrients it is less likely to take place, especially in advanced trainees.

Regulating nutrients along with proper exercise is essential for muscle gain. Muscles grow as a result of working out because intense exercise causes minute tears in the muscle fibers. These are repaired by the body's mechanism so as to withstand a bigger stimulus in future and this expanding of fibers makes the muscles grow in size. This repair happens not while working out but while resting. Therefore proper amounts of nutrients and long hours of rest are a necessity while exercising to gain muscle mass.

It is very common to consider proteins as the sole factor in gaining muscle strength. However, proteins, though vital, are not the only nutrients to be taken care of in your diet. Carbohydrates are just as essential for higher energy required in building up mass. While proteins repair muscles damaged during exercise, the carbohydrate stored in muscles, known as glycogen, acts as the energy store which aids in gaining muscle size. Carbohydrates also kick start many hormonal changes in the body, such as a rise in insulin levels, which favors muscle rebuilding. Unsaturated fats such as olive oil are also essential, because they assist with body processes in relation to muscle gain, and also act as a source of extra calories.

To sum up, effective muscle mass gain without increasing body fat requires precise amounts of nutrients in your diet, effective work outs and sufficient rest. Be a good dieter, but do not blindly follow a diet of restrictions which will ultimately only serve to impair muscle development.

Chapter 5: Beginner's Guide to Flexible Dieting

Even though the idea of flexible dieting sounds appealing, ignorance in the process of tracking macros may dishearten many from embarking on a journey to fitness via flexible dieting. However it is not a difficult task, and this chapter attempts to explain how to count your macro nutrients or utilize applications that help you track down the macros in your food.

Calculating your daily macros is the basis of flexible dieting. However calorie requirement varies from person to person, depending on a variety of factors such as age, metabolism, health condition and lifestyle. The calculated values are only an approximate analysis and are therefore not 100% accurate. However, they provide enough information about one's nutritional requirements to work out a dietary plan.

Calculate your TDEE

Total Daily Energy Expenditure (TDEE) is the required amount of calories per day for normal functioning of the body. This is the amount of calories which are burned in a single day. In order to lose weight, the calorie intake must be less than this value, while it must be more to gain weight. To estimate TDEE, multiply your body weight in pounds to any value from 12-14 depending on your level of activity.

> 12: low activity, people with desk jobs, and no regular exercise

13: medium level activity, someone who does regular exercise

14: highly active, physically engaging job and regular exercise

So, for a moderately active person weighing 190 pounds, the TDEE would be 190lbs x 13= 2,470 Calories.

Counting each macro nutrient is more important than counting calories, because losing weight is different from losing fat.

Each macronutrient has a specific calorie value.

1g Protein = 4 Calories
1g Fat = 9 Calories
1g Carbohydrates = 4 Calories

With these values in mind, one can calculate the ratio of macronutrients.

Protein: Protein is an essential macro nutrient, which is helpful in gaining or maintaining muscle. Your individual protein requirement can be calculated as 1g of protein per pound (if they are heavy lifting) or 0.65 protein per pound of bodyweight. For a 190 pound individual doing weights, it would be 190g x 4 = 760 Calories

Fat: Adjusting the level of fat intake is beneficial in changing body composition. In general, 25% of the total TDEE can be attributed to fat. For a TDEE value of 2,470 Calories,

2470 x 0.25 =617. This divided by 9 which is the calorie value of fat per gram, gives the ratio of fat.
617 divided by 9 = 68.5g Fat

Carbohydrates: carbohydrates are the macros which provide energy for body functions. The remainder of the TDEE value, after estimating values of protein and fat, is assigned to carbohydrates.

For the TDEE of 2,470 Calories, 760 is protein, 617 fat and 1,093 carbohydrates. As 1g carbohydrates is 4 calories, 1,093 divided by 4 gives 273 g as the value of carbohydrates.

The final value of macro nutrients required by a 190 pound individual on a weight training program is 190g protein, 68.5g fat and 273g carbohydrates. Once you have the macronutrient target figured out, you can adjust your food to fit into those values.

A lot of nutritional information will be available on the packaging of food. Read that and determine what is right for you. Make use of a food scale to know the right amount to eat.

In addition you can use an App like My Fitness Pal or Lose It to obtain a customized diet plan to hit your target. They can also scan the bar code to provide nutrient information on any food item. Always try to stay within the guidelines and consistently follow this method to achieve your fitness goals.

Chapter 6: Flexible Dieting is All You Need!

What makes flexible dieting stand out from the scores of other fitness regimes also claiming to be the most suited method for building a better physique? Here's why flexible dieting is the perfect solution to anyone aiming for a bigger, leaner and stronger body.

Having grasped the basics of the relation between nutrition and muscle growth, it's easy to come to the conclusion that eating right is the most imperative factor in bodybuilding or even just in staying fit. Eat wrong and you stay skinny or fat regardless of how much you exercise. Since diet determines 70 to 80% of your body's appearance, it is always a wise decision to pick a diet which will not only enhance your looks, but also make you feel better.

Now, choosing flexible dieting during strength training has a whole load of benefits. It does not require you to spend money on nutrition supplements which are often taken by fitness freaks. There are no feelings of deprivation, as even someone at the peak of their training can allow himself the occasional high fat, low nutrient treat. Lack of fat may often leave you unsatisfied after a meal, even if you have eaten more than your required amount of calories. Adequate amounts of fat are also required to maintain hormone levels like that of testosterone, a reduction of which could affect consumption of calories required for overall muscle gain. Thus, hitting the nutrient target is the best way to bring about changes in body composition.

This is best illustrated by a radical experiment conducted by Professor Mark Haub at Kansas State University, who went on a 'Twinkie diet' which comprised of mostly convenience store food like Twinkies, powdered donuts, Doritos chips, sugary cereals and Oreo biscuits. Although this diet may not be healthy, he lost 27 pounds in two months and his body mass index became a normal 24.9 from his previous 28.8 which is considered overweight. Also, his LDL levels, which are bad cholesterol, reduced by 20% while his good cholesterol, HDL was boosted by 20%. By monitoring his body composition, he was able to bring about changes regardless of the nutritional value of food.

Thus a diet full with nutrients is advisable for gaining or maintaining lean mass. It leads to optimum results by addressing these three points:

- Proteins which help in the preservation of muscles

- Carbohydrates which build up the glycogen stores required for maintaining training intensity

- Healthy fats which help in the synthesis of the various hormones required for muscle growth

Focusing on the right proportions of macro nutrients will help with both muscle build up and loss of fat. It will ensure better performance, faster recovery and help you to stay lean while you bulk. It is also easy to shift from a phase of bulking to cutting or vice versa. There won't be any fat gain during bulking or loss of strength while cutting.

The problem encountered by most body builders is that they may get lean in time for an event or show but will rebound back to gaining pounds as soon as it's over. This happens because the severe deprivation experienced till then leads to over indulgence. On the other hand, getting lean following flexible dieting is not a temporary outcome. There isn't any scope for post show bingeing or losing the hard earned physique in a flexible dieter. That is, this eating practice gets incorporated as a part of your lifestyle, making it easier to adhere to in the long term.

To sum up, understanding the benefits of flexible dieting will help you shape an approach to use nutrition to meet your goals, be it getting bigger and leaner or gaining more body strength. It is the prudent choice for anyone aiming for a better body composition while maintaining a healthy, guilt free relationship with food.

Chapter 7: Why Protein Is So Important

Whatever eating plan you are following, protein is sure to play a big part in it, and rightly so. The thing to remember is that the body needs protein for almost all of its functions, and particularly for building and repairing tissues and cells, but there's more to it than that. Protein helps build healthy bones, muscles and cartilage, as well as helping in the synthesis of enzymes and hormones. So, the body needs protein, but it can't store it, so it requires regular supplies.

Protein and the metabolism

Protein also contains enzymes that help to boost the metabolism. That's important if you're trying to lose weight and/or build muscle. Once it's in the body, before it can do its repair and renewal work, protein has to be converted into a usable form, and this process inevitably burns calories – around 30% of the calories in the protein element of any particular food, in fact. And protein also has to release amino acids, which the body cannot produce alone.

Another great metabolism-boosting function of protein is to build and repair muscle tissue. As well as making your body look more toned and lean on the outside, the protein is doing a great job inside, because muscle burns three times as many calories as fat. While each pound of fat in your body burns just 2 calories a day, a similar amount of muscle burns 6 calories daily. That might not sound much, but if you multiply those 6 calories by your muscle mass, it's going to make a significant difference.

Incorporate plenty of oily fish into your diet too. As well as being high in protein, fish contains Omega-3 fatty acids. As well as having heart healthy properties, these are known to encourage higher levels of calorie burning, which gives a significant boost to the metabolism and helps with fat loss.

Be sure to spread your protein through the day, to keep a steady supply of amino acids coming. This is particularly important in the morning, when the body has had a long break without food sources for energy. It will turn to the muscles for amino acids – since muscles are mostly comprised of protein – rather than going to fat cells for energy. As has already been mentioned, protein, or more accurately the amino acids it contains, is used in almost all bodily processes, and this cannot be obtained from fat stores, so the body – which is self-interested and focused on keeping going – will deplete its muscle stores in the quest for amino acids.

The risks of unbalanced protein consumption

Insufficient protein consumption can result in a number of health and metabolic issues. Apart from loss of muscle mass, people who do not eat enough protein can suffer from insulin resistance, chronic fatigue, loss of skin elasticity and hormone irregularities. This in itself can give rise to potentially serious conditions such as thyroid disease.

Too much protein can also pose problems, although you would have to make a real effort to eat enough to cause health issues. The main concern is that a very high protein diet is also high in saturated fat, which could lease to raised blood cholesterol levels and heart disease. However, too much protein can cause calcium to leach from the bones, leading to loss of bone density and possible osteoporosis in later life.

Choosing healthy proteins

To avoid overdosing on saturated fat, which could block your arteries and cause coronary heart disease, go for lean meat, fish and poultry. Chicken and turkey are good low fat sources of protein, particularly if you discard the skin, where most of the fat is located. Remove visible fat before cooking and eating, and if you need to add extra fat during cooking, keep it to a minimum and go for healthy fats such as olive oil and nut oils.

Legumes, beans, eggs, yogurt, milk and cheese are also good sources of protein. Where possible, go for low fat dairy products to keep down the saturated fat content. Try to include some protein at every meal, so your body has a steady supply through the day. A high protein snack at night – such as a hard-boiled egg, a little cheese or some sliced turkey breast – will help you to feel satisfied so you get a restful night's sleep. This is also important, as that is when the body does the majority of its cell repair and renewal work. This requires so much energy it can only be done when the body is at rest, and this is an important consideration if one of your fitness goals is to build more muscle.

Protein's thermic effect

All food has a thermic effect (TEF). Put simply, that's the energy required to digest what you eat, extract the nutrients and move it through the body. The higher the TEF, the better it is for the metabolism, and the more chance you have of burning off that excess fat. Estimates vary, but protein's TEF is over 20%, compared with around 6% for carbohydrates and 3% for fat.

These figures may not mean much to you, but what you really need to know is that they mean your body has to work harder to digest, convert and transport proteins around your body. That means your metabolism is getting a much-needed boost every time you take a protein hit.

As you can see, protein is very important for a whole lot of reasons. It's necessary for the building and repair of cells, and it's involved in virtually all the body's processes. If you're aiming to burn fat and build lean muscle, protein should be your best friend.

Chapter 8: The Case Against Processed Foods

Theoretically, if you are flexible dieting, you can eat anything you want as long as the macros and calories are fine, right? Theoretically maybe you can, but practically, it would be a very silly and unhealthy thing to do. If you lived on convenience lasagnas, burgers and ice cream, even if your calorie totals and macros were on target, it would be wrong on so many levels.

Macros are only part of the story – you also need micronutrients for healthy body function. That's the vitamins and minerals you get from your food, and the best way to get these micronutrients is from whole, natural foods, not from convenience foods or processed foods. Optimal vitamin content comes from fresh foods ready to eat. Processed foods often have additives to prolong their shelf life and enhance the taste and appearance and these chemicals can interfere with the natural vitamin levels. In addition, keeping products longer than they are naturally intended to be kept before eating is likely to reduce the nutritional content.

Often, synthetic vitamins and minerals are added to processed foods to make up for those nutrients lost during processing. However, when it comes to vitamins and minerals, nothing beats the real thing. The body is designed to use nutrients from food, not from laboratory test tubes, and the plants and animals that feed humans contain innumerable trace elements that are simply not present in manufactured foods. So even if the label says your processed stuff has all the nutrients you need, your body may not see it that way.

The higher your diet is in processed foods, the lower your levels of essential vitamins and nutrients, and that's going to interfere with your objectives of losing fat and building muscle, since muscle needs its nutrients.

As if that weren't enough, processed foods often contain hidden fats and sugars, and extra salt. This is all aimed at improving the appearance, taste and shelf life of the product, but if you ate too many processed foods, you'd be messing about with your macros unless you took the extra ingredients into consideration.

Another problem with processed foods is that very often, they are low in fiber. Fiber is essential for digestive health, as it helps the transit of food through the system and bulks up stools. Without enough fiber, you will be constipated, and that will mess about with your metabolism and impact on fat burning efficiency.

Fiber is also very filling, which is what you want when you're dieting. There's nothing worse than going through the day feeling hungry, and if you make the right food choices, that never needs to happen. Many processed foods fill you up at first, but after a while, you experience a blood sugar dip, and you're hungry again. The fiber in fruits, vegetables and complex carbohydrates helps to keep your blood sugar levels stable and keeps you feeling satisfied until your next meal.

Yet another problem with processed foods – the list just grows, doesn't it? – is that it's possible to get hooked on the flavors of processed food. When that happens, you'll try to replicate those flavors in natural foods. That means you'll start adding more salt and sugar to otherwise healthy foods. Can you see how insidiously processed foods can work their way into every area of your life and diet?

The real killer with processed foods though is the effect they have on your metabolism. The thermic effect of food (TEF) has already been referred to here. That's the amount of energy it takes to process and digest the food that enters your body. Processed foods are designed to be easy and convenient to eat, and that means they are also easy and convenient to digest.

The problem with this is that these foods slip down easily, so you can eat more food in less time. That's a lot more calories in. It takes around 20 minutes to feel full from a meal, which is why having two or three small courses can actually result in eating less food. If food is going down easily, you're going to eat more food in less time, so you won't feel satiated as soon.

Another thing to remember is that it takes less energy in the form of calories to digest a meal made from processed food. In a simple study conducted using cheese sandwiches, the people who ate a wholegrain sandwich made with cheddar cheese used twice as many calories in digesting their snack than the group who ate a sandwich made with processed cheese and white bread. Even though the calorie counts were similar, the wholegrain group felt fuller for longer and expended more calories. With such a dramatic difference in TEF on a single sandwich, imagine what a diet of mainly processed foods would do to your metabolism.

Processed foods are also high in unhealthy trans fats. Trans fats figure a lot in baked goods, because they're cheap and stable at room temperature. However, they are also high in Omega-6 fatty acids, which counteract the good work antioxidants do in the body and also contribute to internal inflammation. Internal inflammation contributes to many chronic conditions such as diabetes, heart disease, arthritis and obesity, so trans fats should be avoided if you're trying to stay healthy, lose weight and build muscle.

You won't find trans fats in whole foods – even saturated fats are healthier than trans fats, which may appear on ingredient panels as 'hydrogenated oils.' Check out the labels next time you go grocery shopping – you'll be surprised how many foods contain these unhealthy fats.

If you're not convinced by now that processed foods are unhealthy, and have no place in flexible dieting, maybe this will tip the balance. Processed foods increase the risk factors for obesity, diabetes, heart disease and hypertension. Hardly the way to get lean and build muscle, is it?

Chapter 9: Weight Loss And Fat Loss Are Different

When people talk about losing weight, what they really want to lose is fat. Everything in your body obviously weighs something. For example, the human head, complete with brain, weighs around 10 lbs. So if you cut off your head – or somebody else cut it off for you – you could say you'd lost 10 lbs in weight. Well, you couldn't, because you'd be dead. Cutting your head off is not a healthy way to lose weight.

If you go on a strict diet, you will also lose weight, but a lot of that weight will be down to losing water in the first few days of a strict diet. When you start to eat more normally, that water weight loss will come right back at you, with maybe a few more pounds for good measure. Really, when you say you want to lose weight, what you really mean is you want to lose fat.

The percentage of fat to lean body mass (LBM) varies, depending on your sex, your level of activity and the condition of your body. Athletes may have as little as 10% fat against LBM, so the total body fat of a 150 lb male would be 15 lbs. However, someone who is morbidly obese could have as much as 40 – 50% of body fat. A 200 lb woman may well have 100 lbs of fat, and if that woman goes on a weight loss diet, it's really that fat she's targeting and hoping to lose, so maybe it's time to tidy up the thinking and say what you really mean.

Thinking in terms of fat loss sits better with the principles of flexible dieting too. Flexible dieting is all about focusing on what goes into your body so you get the body you want. In order to do that, and realize why previous diets have failed. Put simply, it's because you've concentrated on losing weight, rather than directing your energies towards losing fat. Sounds simple put like that, doesn't it?

In some ways it is. What you're aiming for is LBM, so what you want to get rid of is your fat mass, which can be anything between 10% and 50% of your body weight, according to expert opinion. Humans are better programmed to hang on to body fat rather than lose it as a failsafe against starvation, which is why the metabolism slows down when you restrict the food supply. So it's difficult to lose weight, as the body tries to hang on to its fat stores. But because there was no real danger of getting fat in the distant past of human evolution, there is no corresponding mechanism to prevent weight gain.

Even when and if you manage to lose weight on a diet, your body will remember the lean times, and once you start to increase your calorie intake, the body will hang on to those calories and convert them to fat cells for future insurance against lean times. So a better strategy is, rather than embark on drastic dietary changes – 'going on' a diet, make small but significant changes that can be sustained over time. You won't see a significant weight loss, but there will be fat loss of perhaps 1 lb a week.

Chapter 10: Changing Your Attitude Towards Dieting

The main reason so many diets fail is that people take an 'all or nothing' approach. They'll stick rigidly to the diet for however long – a week, two weeks, a month, maybe more. Then one day they would kill for a cookie, so they resist for a while, but the craving gets stronger. The cookie is calling, and not just a single cookie either – the whole packet is crying 'Eat me, for the love of God!' and before you know it, the packet has disappeared, and at least 1,000 calories have attached themselves to your daily total.

So what do you do? You junk the diet because you've 'failed.' You've forgotten the week or more that you've stuck with the diet, eating and drinking exactly what you should. All you can focus on is the moment of madness – or rather those few minutes of madness – that saw you demolish all those cookies and all those calories. So, you come off the diet, because you've just ruined it.

Actually, you haven't ruined it – yet. But you're going to, because you'll use that lapse as an excuse to forget all about dieting. You may tell yourself you're meant to be fat, or that you don't have the willpower to stick to a diet, or any manner of other things. And you'll be generating a self-fulfilling prophecy, because that few minutes of bingeing will probably lead to weeks or even months of eating what you want, until you've gained all the weight you lost, and a few pounds more for good measure.

Flexible dieting is different. Your whole approach to dieting is different, because you understand how calories work, and you understand how your body works. You know that no way could that one little lapse scupper all the good work of the past weeks, so you put it behind you and move on, looking at it logically.

So what if you just ate an extra 1,000 calories. It's one lapse in a week, which works out to about an extra 150 calories each day. Even leaving the 1,000 calories as a unit, you need to eat 3,500 extra calories more than your body needs for normal function to gain one pound. At worst, your cookie chomp has gained about 5 ounces. But what if you got up and went for a walk or a swim right now? That could mitigate at least half of those calories.

That's the big difference with flexible dieting. You look at the big picture, instead of being blinkered and just seeing a failure to stick to the diet. With flexible dieting, you can compensate before and after the event, as calories are planned on a week by week basis. Or you can just say, 'So I ate a few cookies, it's not the end of the world or of my diet,' and move on, without regret.

The reason you can do that is because you realize that flexible dieting is for the long term, and results matter over the long term, not a few weeks of some diet or other. Because you're looking at the bigger picture, you can be rational about it all. What you do in the space of a few mad minutes doesn't really matter one way or the other, but what is important is how you plan your meals and activities over the course of a month. If Cookiegate was your only lapse, it won't have impacted on your fat loss. In fact by shocking your system with an overload of food, the slight rise in metabolism might even compensate a little for that.

Give yourself permission to deviate from the diet occasionally – it's called flexible dieting after all. And when you do deviate – which ironically may not happen too often now you've allowed yourself to do it – you can enjoy your treat in the knowledge that you are in control of what you eat and when. Giving yourself permission to take a short break from the healthy eating can be very empowering. Instead of seeing yourself a failure – which was what happened in the scenario described above – you know that you are a person who is so confident of success in reaching their fat loss and fitness goals they can be relaxed about sticking rigidly to the guidelines of the diet.

Another way in which attitudes to dieting need to change is when the leash is slackened for a while and you have a free meal or structured re-feed. These used to be called 'cheat meals' and 'cheat days,' and they still are in some places, but people tend to apply negative connotations to the word 'cheat,' so it's not a phrase you hear as often as previously.

In the case of flexible dieting, the word 'cheat' is particularly inappropriate. The diet is flexible, so how can you cheat, when there are no forbidden foods? Again, it's a question of short term diet syndrome. You're following a diet, so you have to eat what's on the diet, and nothing more. If you're on course with your macro units, and you've been sticking to the diet and exercising for several weeks, why not have a free meal or a structured re-feed? If you time it right, and don't use the occasion as an excuse to overload your body with all kinds of junk food, or as many calories as you can muster, it can give you a nice little boost if your fat loss stalls, or simply if you feel you deserve a break from the dieting.

It's all about the attitude. Flexible dieting is really flexible, so you need to focus on the idea that dieting doesn't need to be absolute. It's okay to eat something you don't think you should be eating, because no foods are forbidden. And if you give into temptation and eat more than you really should, hey, everyone is human, so don't beat yourself up over it, and certainly don't ditch the diet because of it. On the contrary, enjoy your treat and savor it – this is a long term plan, and everyone deserves the odd treat. It's not going to break the calorie bank, or undo weeks of good work, so just enjoy the moment, then move on without fuss or guilt. Tomorrow is another day, after all.

Chapter 11: The Right Approach To Free Meals And Structured Re-feeds

Free meals and structured re-feeds are breaks in the dieting pattern. A free meal is basically a meal where you eat what you fancy, and don't bother tracking the macros. You may want to save this for a special occasion or a celebration, like Thanksgiving or a birthday or anniversary. A structured re-feed is something different altogether. It's a deliberate strategy of overloading on carbohydrates for several hours or even a full day while still tracking macros. Both free meals and re-feeds are thought to provide a metabolic boost after a few weeks of dieting by switching around the way you eat and taking more calories on board. This also has a hormonal effect which can be helpful in fat burning.

At one time, they were known as cheat meals and cheat days, and indeed they are still referred to as such in some quarters, but people tend to attach negative connotations to the word 'cheat,' so it's not as widely used as previously. Free meals and re-feeds have psychological as well as physical benefits. The thought of being able to eat what you like, or overloading on carbs after several weeks of deprivation can be very motivational, making people feel less deprived and more relaxed. Even on a flexible diet, there comes a time when you just feel like a break, and free meals and re-feeds allow that to happen, while serving a useful purpose at the same time.

Benefits of free meals

Perhaps the main benefit of a free meal is that it allows you to eat what you want, in the quantities you want. No calorie counting or macro tracking – just eat and enjoy. They say a little of what you fancy does you good, and that's the main benefit of a free meal. If you've been craving a particular food or cuisine, now's the time to indulge it. You'll enjoy the freedom, then return to your diet the next day with renewed motivation. At least, that's the idea!

Another advantage is that the calorie hike entailed in a free meal revs up the metabolism slightly, and stimulates hormonal activity. This can boost fat burning for several hours afterwards. If you incorporate two free meals a week, this can make a significant difference to the metabolic rate.

The free meal gives you a break from tracking, as well as a break from dieting. It's the freedom to enjoy what you want, in the quantities you want, without worrying about calorie content or nutrient proportions. It's like a mini break from dieting, and the longer you've been dieting, the more you'll appreciate it. Because the break is planned, there is no guilt attached to eating foods which normally don't figure in your eating plan.

Disadvantages of free meals

Everything has its cons as well as the pros, and the major disadvantage of free meals is that you need to have a certain amount of control if you're not going to go off on a huge binge. That's not the name of the game. A free meal should be pretty much like any other meal. Don't head for the all you can eat buffet, because that's too much of a temptation to totally pig out.

Another problem is the risk of overeating, which could make you feel uncomfortable and bloated for the remainder of the day. That could take some of the enjoyment away from the fact of just having eaten a free meal containing all the foods you love.

Getting it right

Plan your free meal so that you get maximum enjoyment from it – make it an occasion. You may want to eat out for your free meal, or have friends around for tapas or a dinner party. In some ways, the restaurant option is best, because then there will be an element of portion control which regulates the scope for overindulging. Don't even consider an all you can eat buffet – unless you are like Superman and have a will of steel.

Evenings are probably the best time for your free meal. It makes it more of an occasion, and it's a good way to round off the day before returning to the diet proper tomorrow. Also, if the free meal is earlier in the day, you may find it difficult to get back on track.

Basically, you should treat your free meal as an ordinary meal with a few little extras. Don't try to set up a record for cramming in as much as you possible can within the time frame, and try to have some healthy choices on your plate. It certainly shouldn't be a processed food fest – try to stick with natural foods, but allow yourself the luxury of rich sauces if you want them, and larger portions. Above all, enjoy your free meal – take the time to savor each mouthful, and enjoy your break from dieting.

You can probably incorporate two free meals into your diet each week without compromising your fat loss. However, it's not a good idea to implement free meals in the first weeks of any new diet. Get used to the eating plan, and start losing fat, so you're motivated to get straight back into the diet after your free meal. If you're struggling to adapt to the diet, a free meal might send you off the rails, and that's not the idea at all.

A free meal is a welcome break from the routine of dieting, not a get out clause. You should be sure you're into the swing of healthy eating and well motivated first.

Benefits of structured re-feeds

Structured re-feeds can last from a few hours to 24 hours. Some fitness experts say around 5 hours is long enough, while others recommend a full day. It's down to personal preference, and also self-control. The big advantage of a structured re-feed is that it tops up glycogen levels in the muscles – that's the carbohydrate stores that give strength to the muscles. A re-feed also prevents loss of LBM, pretty much forcing the body to burn fat stores again. Generally speaking, if supplies of energy are low, the body will store the fat cells and get its energy from muscles. Re-feeding halts that process.

Loading up on carbs also helps to balance the hormones so the metabolism works more effectively, so a re-feed is a good strategy to take on board, provided it's done right. It also improves insulin sensitivity, which helps guard against diabetes and also helps the muscles to make the most effective use of proteins. If you're aiming for lean, sculpted muscles, a re-feed can help with this.

Disadvantages of structured re-feeds

If you're going to do a structured re-feed, you need a certain amount of self-control if you're not going to go off on a mega binge. Alternatively, some people may interpret 'Eat lots of carbs' as 'Fill up on junk food.' In fact, you should be filling up on healthy, complex carbohydrates. You should only attempt a structured re-feed if you are really committed to dieting and fat loss.

Some people who are particularly sensitive to eating large amounts of carbohydrates may become drowsy due to the release of serotonin after a large carb intake. This phenomenon is known as 'carb coma.'

Getting it right

It's even more important to get a structured re-feed right than a free meal. That's because there's the potential to take on board a lot of extra calories over a fairly long period of time. You need to be sensible about this – a 24 hour re-feed doesn't mean starting to eat just after midnight and keeping going until almost midnight. That way lies trouble.

It's not all about the carbs either. You still need to take on board some lean protein and healthy fruits and vegetables for fiber. Otherwise, you're likely to feel sluggish. However, because you are loading on the carbs, you can enjoy some of the sweeter, high carbohydrate and high calorie treats that you may have passed up on your diet.

Keep your fat consumption low on re-feed days – aim for less than 50 grams. Too much fat will see you regaining the body fat you tried so hard to lose. A structured re-feed needs careful tracking, to ensure you get the macros right, so spend some time working out your menu – don't just shovel in the carbs as if they're going out of fashion.

Spread your eating over the period of the re-feed, aiming to eat something every 2 – 3 hours rather than going for a big blow out which will probably make you feel very sluggish every 4 – 5 hours. As for carb quantities, start with around 1.5 grams per pound of LBM, working up to 3 – 4 grams if you tolerate it well. There are numerous calculators online to help you to do this, or you can ask a personal trainer or a bodybuilding friend. They'll be able to advise on this.

One word of warning – if you normally have two free meals a week, replace one of them with the re-feed, otherwise you'll be taking in far too many carbs and calories. Also, it's not a good idea to have more than two deviant diet days in a week. You could get out of the dieting mindset.

Structured re-feeding isn't a good fit for everyone. If you normally follow a low carbohydrate, high protein diet, and feel good on it, a re-feed might make you feel fatigued and sluggish, due to the high carb content. It doesn't have to form part of your flexible dieting routine, but if it suits your mindset and your style of eating, it does have a number of physical and psychological advantages.

Chapter 12: Taking a Dieting Break

Flexible dieting allows for taking a break when you need to. That could be a planned break for a vacation or holiday period, or an unplanned break, maybe because something comes up that makes dieting difficult. A business trip at short notice, perhaps, or an unscheduled visit for a family crisis.

When such a situation arises, it's easier to take a break from the diet for a number of reasons. If you're on vacation, or celebrating over Christmas, why put yourself through the ordeal of watching everyone else relax and enjoy good food while you're tracking your macros? Yes, a flexible diet allows you to eat much more – well, flexibly, than most diets, but you can't relax completely if you're still tracking your macros and counting calories.

As long as you've been dieting for at least a few weeks, and have been losing fat and building lean muscle, you can afford a one or two week break, without having to worry about undoing all your good work. The worst that can happen is that you might regain a pound or two of fat, but it will soon disappear again when you get back on track.

And if the break is unplanned, for whatever reason, there may be an element of stress involved, or hard work and long hours with no chance to exercise or plan your meals. So it makes sense to take a dieting break for a week or two. If possible, keep it to no longer than two weeks, because any longer and it may be difficult to get back into the dieting groove.

Handled properly, a dieting break, whether planned or unplanned, can be good both physically and psychologically. In addition, its good training for the time when you've reached your goals of fat loss and muscle building, and you can move from flexible dieting to weight and body composition maintenance. However, maybe that's getting ahead of the game a little. So, how do you go about taking a break from flexible dieting?

First of all, don't even consider it until you've been dieting for at least a couple of months, if not more. Think of those comedians who make a sketch – or even a career – about playing the piano badly, or doing magic tricks badly. The reason they are so funny is that in order to play the piano or conjure hilariously badly, they need to be able to do those things well in the first place. The same principle applies with flexible dieting. In order to take a successful break, you need to thoroughly understand the main concepts of the diet. You need to be confident in your approach to fat loss and muscle building – so confident that you don't worry about taking a break, whether planned or unplanned.

The free meal diet break

A simple way of taking a diet break would be to eat breakfast and lunch, together with any snacks, as you've been doing all along, then have a free meal at night. If you've been flexible dieting for a while, chances are you've settled into a routine where breakfast and lunch follow a similar pattern of maybe four or five choices in rotation, with your favorite standby snacks in between. You're so used to these choices, you don't even need to track the macros any more.

Many people – whether on diets or not – seem to have favorites they rotate for breakfast and lunch. It's the evening meals where the variation occurs, and if you're flexible dieting, that's where you need to keep track of those macros. Making each evening meal a free meal gives you a taste of the best of both worlds – your daytime eating is controlled, but without the hassle of tracking macros and calories, and in the evening, you can relax and enjoy whatever takes your fancy.

The advantage of doing it this way is that, by eating 'on plan' all day, you're limiting the margin for splurging, because just that one meal is totally free. If you're a bit wary of taking a diet break, maybe this mix of diet meals and free meals is the best fit for you.

Okay, you may gain a little over the course of the break, but it shouldn't become unmanageable or disheartening, and a week back in full diet mode should sort out any gains. If you've been dieting for a while, you may have reached a plateau where you're not burning fat any more. That's because your metabolism has adjusted to your diet. As has been mentioned before, your body doesn't know the difference between planned starvation in the form of a diet, and starvation because there is no food available.

Why take a diet break?

Ever heard the saying 'If it ain't broke, don't fix it?' Maybe you're asking that question right now. If the diet is going well, why take a break anyway? If you're committed to it, surely you can tweak it to fit any situations? Well, sometimes you need to step away from a situation. Vacations and stress or emergencies are just two of them, or it may simply be a physical thing.

Serial dieters often get problems with the metabolism, as it switches to survival mode when the supplies of food stop coming. And even if this is your first diet, or your first successful diet, where you're actually losing fat and building muscle so you're radically changing your body composition, you will hit this particular wall at some point.

Changing the way you eat by taking a diet break will give the metabolism a kick and stabilize the body's hormones so that it can start burning fat stores again. As was mentioned in the chapter on structured re-feeds, when the body needs energy, it doesn't automatically take it from fat stores – those are the insurance policy against the lean times. The body takes its essential energy from the muscles, thus breaking down the tissues and undoing your hard work.

When the eating habits change and the perceived threat of starvation has passed, the metabolism returns to its normal rate, and the fat burning process starts again. The human body is a precision machine, and when it believes all is well with its world and there is an adequate supply of food, it returns to default mode, which is basically keeping the body at a healthy weight, and in the best condition to fight or flee from threats.

If you have fat to lose, the metabolism will help you do that, as long as it feels it is getting adequate nutrition, and that's why rigid, very low calorie diets will never really help you get rid of body fat. However, although taking a break from a flexible diet might result in a small fat gain, this should be well compensated for by the faster fat burning that happens as a result of the metabolism boost.

The free meal diet break is probably the easiest way to go about scaling back the diet, by revving up the metabolism and drawing emotional strength and motivation from a relaxation of your diet regime. You could also just let everything go hang and eat what you want, and unless you were really greedy and ate everything in sight, you'd be unlikely to gain a lot of fat. Enjoy your sabbatical, and come back refreshed and raring to go in the fight against fat.

Chapter 13: Why Eating Lower Fat Content Matters

Throughout this book you will have seen several references to low fat eating. Maybe it's given you pause for thought. After all, this is flexible dieting, and doesn't that mean eating what you want? Well, to some extent it does, but flexible dieting is also all about the macros. That's the three major food groups: proteins, carbohydrates and fats.

Of the three groups, fats are seen as the bad guys. They have more calories per gram for a start. Proteins and carbohydrates contain just 4 calories per gram, while fats contain more than double that amount at 9 calories. That should give you pause for thought if nothing else does. But when you examine just what happens to fat when it enters the body, that is a real eye opener.

People can easily eat more high fat foods than other foods, without even noticing. That's because high fat foods seem to slip down easier and taste nicer, so you don't realize how much you're actually eating. There's a fancy scientific name for this – it's called passive over consumption. So now you know. Passive over consumption is not like eating too much of anything else. You don't get that feeling of bloating and 'Can't eat another thing,' so you keep on eating. You'll know what this means if you've ever sat down with a party sized bag of chips and emptied it before you even realized it. You'll have taken in a load of calories, but you don't feel full, as if you couldn't eat another thing. In fact, it there was another bag of chips going, you'd probably get stuck into those as well.

Unlike protein and fiber, fat doesn't satisfy your hunger or regulate the amount of food you're likely to eat at a meal or at the buffet table. So you're going to eat more calories if you're eating high fat foods. Remember fat contains twice as many calories per gram as protein or carbohydrates. And your body doesn't have to put in the same work chewing and digesting high fat foods as you do with protein and carbohydrates. That means your metabolism isn't working so hard, so not only are you taking in a double dose of calories, you're not offsetting the intake by burning extra calories to digest and process the food.

It follows then that if you limit the fats in your diet, you'll also automatically reduce the number of calories you're consuming. However, if you lower the fat content too much, your diet may start to look unimaginative and uninteresting, so you need to strike a happy balance. Nutrition experts are now recommending that a diet which is moderate in fat, with about 25% of daily calories coming from fat, is more effective in fat burning than a very low fat diet.

Everyone needs a certain amount of fat for health, but some fats are just not healthy, and they should be avoided. Trans fats are a good case in point here. Trans fats are hydrogenated vegetable oils which are added to prepared convenience meals to improve appearance and taste and extend shelf life. However they are also linked to several chronic health conditions, such as heart disease, diabetes and internal inflammation, which contributes to a whole lot more. You can avoid trans fats by avoiding processed food, because that's where you mainly find them.

Trans fats are basically hydrogenated oils – they don't occur naturally, they have to undergo a process to get that unhealthy. That's yet another reason for avoiding processed foods, if you really needed one.

Saturated fats come from animal protein, so unless you're a vegetarian or vegan, you can't avoid them altogether. There's nothing wrong with a little saturated fat though – everyone needs some fat for health, but the problems arise when people forget to apply that word moderation and pig out on steaks the size of a small country on a regular basis. That's when your arteries start getting blocked and you pile on the weight, in effect almost begging for a heart attack.

Flexible dieting advocates eating lean protein for a number of very good reasons. It keeps you feeling satisfied for longer, the body has to work harder to process protein, so it uses more calories and burns more fat, and protein is needed for building lean muscle and a host of other internal processes.

That's why you'll always see the exhortation to eat 'lean protein.' That's fish, egg whites, poultry and lean red meat. Beans and pulses also contain protein, but animal protein is more easily and effectively used by the body. You can make your protein even healthier by trimming off visible fat before serving and cooking. At 9 calories a gram, even a small amount of fat trimmed from that steak – regular sized of course – can make a difference to your calorie count and your overall health.

The healthiest fat of all is monounsaturated fat. That's what you find in olive oil, and it's just about the best you can put into your body. It's at the heart of the Mediterranean Diet, which is reckoned by experts all over the world to be the healthiest diet going. Despite a predilection for wine, saturated fat and rich sauces, the French have a lower incidence of heart disease than many other countries. It's the same in Spain, where vegetarianism is an alien concept and saturated fat is served up at every meal. Both countries have more smokers than average too, yet they are still healthier than many developed countries, with fewer deaths from heart disease, diabetes and cancer.

Experts put that down to the Mediterranean Diet, which isn't really a diet at all, rather a way of eating which is really healthy. Other factors are involved, such as no processed food, lots of fish for heart-healthy Omega-3 fatty acids and plenty of fresh vegetables laden with fiber and antioxidants. However, the cornerstone of the diet is olive oil, and Mediterranean countries use it like it's going out of fashion tomorrow.

Flexible dieting advocates moderation, so nobody would suggest you glug out the olive oil, but it's worth making it your number one, default fat. Use it for shallow frying, and in marinades and dressings. The healthiest version of this very healthy oil is extra virgin first cold pressing, since that has gone through less processing than other incarnations of olive oil. Use it whenever you need to use oil, and even spread it on bread instead of butter. That's something else the Mediterranean people do – they don't get the British and American fascination with putting butter on bread. They use it, but only in cooking for a richer flavor than olive oil can provide. It's worth taking that lesson to keep your fats under control.

How much fat should you be taking in each day? If you're looking to keep under 50 grams, which is one recommendation, aim for no more than 4 tablespoons of oil a day. There will also be some residual fat in your proteins – particularly red meat, which has a marbling of fat to provide the flavor. That's why it's important to go for lean meat and remove any visible fat. Go for extra lean ground beef to keep down the fat content, as it's more difficult to remove it, although you can skim off some of the fat as the meat cooks. Don't be too stringent though – take out all the fat and you take out a lot of the flavor. That's one of the reasons people don't stick with low fat diets – they're often so low in fat that they're too darned bland to enjoy.

It's not difficult to eat low fat if you have a little knowledge of nutrition, avoid processed food and make sensible, healthy choices. As well as keeping the calorie count down so that the body is forced to burn its fat stores, low fat eating is also a kind of insurance policy against heart disease, obesity and other chronic conditions in later life. What's not to love about low fat eating when it's part of a flexible, satisfying diet?

Chapter 14: Carbohydrates and Insulin

All carbohydrates are not created equal, neither are they the Spawn of Satan, as some low carb diet advocates would have you believe. Because carbohydrates are closely linked to insulin, and insulin is closely linked to blood sugar spikes, increased appetite and diabetes, there's a perceived view in some quarters that carbohydrates make you fat and/or give you diabetes. That's a gross oversimplification, and it's a prejudiced and slanderous view of the relationship between carbs and insulin. It's almost like saying that if your brother is a homicidal maniac, it follows that you must be one too, purely based on that close relationship.

The thing is, insulin gets a bad press because of its relationship to diabetes and carbs. More of the murderous family thing. In fact, insulin does a lot of good in the body when it's managed well. It helps to preserve muscle and pull fat from the blood, so it's a real friend to the flexible dieter. Most things work better as a team, and insulin and carbohydrates are no exception. Managed right, they can be a great combination.

Insulin helps stop the body from using glycogen stores in the muscles while you're dieting, so effectively it's preserving and even building muscles, since it also plays a part in sending amino acids to the muscles. Since flexible dieting is all about building muscle and burning fat, you need insulin to do what it does best, and to do that, insulin needs carbohydrates, and plenty of them. It's a necessary part of the process of digesting carbs.

And a number of studies show that in the short term, while a low carb diet can help with initial weight loss, over the long term, there is very little difference. The thing is, whatever name a diet goes by – low carb, low fat, Atkins, South Beach, the Zone, even the Cabbage Soup Diet – it works because you take in fewer calories than you expend. Even if you don't appear to be counting calories, the diet is designed to do it for you. You could live off Big Macs, and as long as you ate less calories than your body used, you'd lose weight. You'd feel foul and your body composition would be less than perfect, but you'd lose weight.

That's the thing with most diets – they focus on weight loss rather than fat loss and muscle gain. As mentioned previously, there's no quick and easy way of knowing whether the weight you lose is water, fat, muscle or a combination of all three. The only way you can be sure to get the body you really want is to follow a diet designed to build muscle and force the body to burn fat rather than raid the muscles for energy. And that sort of diet is necessarily high in carbs and proteins, due to the special relationship between carbs, insulin and amino acids.

Carbohydrates are important energy providers, they help to keep you feeling full for longer and they help to build lean muscle. As one of the three macronutrients along with proteins and fats, carbs are an important element of flexible dieting, so it's worth taking the time to get both the type of carbs you eat and the quantities right.

There are two kinds of carbohydrates – refined and complex. Refined carbs are those which have been processed, sometimes heavily, like white bread, flour, rice and pasta. Complex carbs have been through less processing, if any, and are closer to their natural state – whole foods effectively.

High carb diets don't suit everybody, though. Everyone is different, due to body composition, genetic inheritance and the way their body processes nutrients. While some people feel really well on a diet high in carbohydrates, others may get hungry and experience fluctuations in energy levels and slow weight loss, or even weight gain.

For example, insulin sensitive people – that's those whose bodies make the best use of insulin – do well on high carb diets, often losing as much as twice the amount of weight as people on low carb diets, especially when they have a lot to lose. However, people who are insulin resistant – where the body produces insulin but is unable to use it effectively for various reasons – are likely to lose more weight on a low carb diet.

How can you tell which category you fall into without taking tests? Well, if you're insulin sensitive, and your body is using the insulin it produces as Nature intended, you'll feel and look good on a high carb diet. You'll be mentally alert, your muscles will feel strong and healthy, and you'll have plenty of energy, as well as feeling satisfied by your diet. In other words, you're ready to rock, big time.

On the other hand, if you are insulin resistant, you're likely to feel very different on a high carb diet. Think bloating, wind (not the kite-flying type) lethargy and feeling hungry soon after eating. Not good is it? And you may not be sleeping well either, which is why you feel so drained. For you, a low carb diet may be a better fit.

Until you try, though, you won't know, so don't let the Low Carb Kings blind you to the real science of how carbohydrates can help you to lose body fat and build muscle at the same time.

Chapter 15: Why Flexible Dieting Works When Other Diets Fail

The world is full of people who have tried – and failed – to lose weight. Most of them have done it many times – they are serial dieters, and while they can and do lose weight – often in large amounts and very quickly – they often regain it again at the end of the diet, with a little more for good measure. Why does that happen? Because they 'go on' a diet to lose weight, then 'come off' it when they reach their goal.

They probably follow the diet religiously – if they didn't they wouldn't lose the weight in the first place. However, what they fail to do is learn long term healthy eating habits. They see a diet as a temporary thing to get rid of a few extra pounds, and a sort of penance for eating everything they want to eat. Dieting is collateral damage limitation, whereas it should be a permanent commitment to a healthy lifestyle. Not so much a diet, more a healthy eating plan for life.

If the thought of dieting for life has sent you rushing for a super size pizza, just get right back here! A diet for life is only going to work if it's sustainable and satisfying, and that's where flexible dieting wins out over all the other methods. It's not really dieting as such, because it builds a firm foundation for healthy eating for life.

Flexible dieting is consistent – the principles are the same whether you're trying to lose fat, build muscle, maintain a healthy weight or add bulk, maybe for competitions, or just to look better in the skin you're in. It's estimated that around 95% of dieters fail to get weight off and keep it off because when one diet fails, they try another, and another, always with the same results. The weight comes off, and then it goes back on again when they come off the diet.

Flexible dieting is a whole lifestyle, because it's a long term approach to nutrition and building the body you want, and you're in control at every stage of the process. You can take breaks as and when you need to, either as free meals, scheduled re-feeds or total diet breaks, either planned or impromptu, depending on circumstances. No other diet gives you so much freedom, or places so much trust and confidence in the hands of the dieter. While this may seem a little scary at first, the end result is that you learn all about nutrition, how it works generally and more importantly, how it works as applied to your body and your circumstances.

Everybody is different, and every body is unique – that's something most diet plans fail to take into consideration. They are 'one size fits all' diets, and the problem is, one size rarely fits all, as you will realize if you've ever bought a cheap dress or shirt from the market. It looks okay on the hanger – just as the diets look okay on the website or on paper. However, when you try to fit it to you as an individual, it doesn't always work out, and you are inevitably disappointed.

Flexible dieting is different, because it's – well, flexible! The macros are based on your nutritional needs, weight and calorie count. All diets come down to calorie count in the end – to lose a pound in weight, or more precisely fat, you need to take in 3,500 calories less than your body needs to keep going on a daily basis. That principle applies whether the diet is low fat, low carb, high protein, vegetarian or meal replacement. It may not be obvious that you are counting calories, but in some way, shape or form, that's exactly what you're doing, because if you weren't, you wouldn't be losing weight. You need to accept that.

You can design your diet to fit your lifestyle, circumstances and nutritional needs. If you are insulin sensitive and can make efficient use of the insulin your body produces, you will do well on a high carbohydrate diet. However, if carbs make you sluggish and lacking in energy to the point where you feel too weak to exercise, chances are you are insulin resistant, and a low carb diet may be a better fit. With flexible dieting, you are in the driving seat, and you make that decision, based on your body's response to the fuel – that is food – you put into it, and the results you get out of it.

It's a bit like filling your car at the gas station – if you don't use the best fuel for your motor, you'll lose out on performance and may even do permanent damage to the engine. The same goes for your body. You need to find the best diet for you, at any given time.

The proportions of the fuel you put into your body will depend on several factors – metabolism, body composition, genetic disposition, activity and fitness levels. It can't be stressed enough that everyone is different. Some people only need to look at a calorie to pile on weight, while others can pig out on all sorts and maintain a lean body. That may have a lot to do with genetics – some people are more predisposed to weight gain than others, and it tends to run in families.

The metabolism is the big thing to deal with, because it thinks it knows best what your body needs, and generally, it does. However, to the metabolism, a diet is a starvation threat, so it slows down to conserve energy and keep you alive. It hasn't caught up with the times, and it doesn't realize you are never going to starve unless you're locked in a room with no food and water. Most diets don't allow for this, but flexible dieting is geared for this natural phenomenon with the inclusion of free meals and scheduled re-feeds, as well as dieting breaks, designed to rev up the metabolism by changing the way you eat temporarily.

With most diets, that would cause panic stations, because the likely gain of a pound or two during a break would be seen as a Very Bad Thing. However, flexible dieting is not centered around the scales, so the attitude is different. If a short break means a slight gain in weight, but better fat burning subsequently, it's the right thing to do. Flexible dieting focuses on the bigger picture.

That's the main reason why flexible dieting works where other diets fail. It's not a blinkered approach, so it's easily adaptable to changes in circumstances and body composition. No time to prepare healthy meals, or too stressed to keep your mind on the diet? Take a break, and come back refreshed and newly motivated. Vacation coming up? Give the diet a vacation too and enjoy a relaxing break with good food and good company. Fancy a pizza for dinner? Go ahead – just factor it into your macros. Nothing is forbidden in flexible dieting, and that, dear reader, is why it succeeds when all other diets fail.

Conclusion

Flexible dieting is a great way to lose weight, and it can help you on your journey towards a bigger, leaner and stronger body. However, you need to take a sensible approach to nutrition. While no foods are forbidden on the plan, you will obtain maximum fat burning and muscle building benefits by eating protein at every meal and ensuring that you eat plenty of fresh, natural foods which contain the micronutrients your body needs.

It's also important to understand how the metabolism works, so that you can time your meals to keep it working all the time, and choose foods which make the body work harder in order to digest them. This keeps the metabolism elevated and helps burn fat more quickly.

The next step is to take the information and suggestions from this book and apply them to your daily life. Don't wait until tomorrow, apply what you've learned today while it's still fresh in your mind. Determine what's important to you and your fitness goals, calculate the macro nutrient levels applicable to reach those goals, use some of the helpful tips from this book, then work your Ass off to reach the **ultimate you!**

Preview of My Other Books

If you are interested in improving your health then you may also be interested in one of my other books "Bodyweight Training: Lose Weight, Build Muscle, Get Lean - The No B.S. Approach to Bodyweight Strength Training"

If you want to be strong, lean and muscular fast without steroids or wasting ridiculous amounts of time in the gym... then you will want to read this book

How would you like to burn fat, improve overall stamina, strength, energy, agility, coordination and balance whilst losing weight and building muscle to achieve a naturally sculptured awesome looking body? If so then welcome to your new journey into the life of calisthenics!!!

The great news about calisthenics exercises is that they are completely FREE and relatively easy to perform. You don't need an expensive gym membership or expensive equipment as all the exercises can be performed at home using your own body weight. Exercises can be performed by people in all age groups and genders without risk of injury when performed properly.

You can get this book today on Amazon by following this link:

www.amazon.com/Fitness-Bodyweight-Training-Approach-bodyweight-ebook/dp/B00XRCBAPC

Or alternatively you can go to my Author Bio page on Amazon here:

www.amazon.com/Chris-Cole/e/B00Q1D4RDQ

www.ingramcontent.com/pod-product-compliance
Lightning Source LLC
Chambersburg PA
CBHW070815290526
45795CB00002B/725